Table of Contents

Introduction

Inflammation is a natural, protective response to infection. Its purpose is to remove pathogens or damaged tissue, although it's very important that the location of damage is carefully monitored. If inflammation persists longer than needed, it can cause harm to the body. Inflammatory disease atherosclerosis, also known as coronary artery disease (CAD), is a very common contributing factor to life-threatening heart conditions including strokes and heart attacks.

Atherosclerosis, most often through thrombosis, leads to ischemic heart disease and ischemic stroke, the leading causes of death and disability worldwide. Advanced atherosclerosis and imaging of atherosclerosis are the focus of this dissertation with particular emphasis on the vulnerable plaque and vulnerable plaque detection. In this thesis, aspects of advanced atherosclerosis and the vulnerable plaque in humans are first introduced. Then the basis for the selected animal models and methods used are described. Hereafter, the aims of the dissertation are formulated.

ISCHEMIC HEART DISEASE

Worldwide, ischemic heart disease is the leading cause of death and more people die from ischemic heart disease in low and middle-income countries than in high-income countries.

In ischemic heart disease, the heart suffers from ischemia (Greek: isch- restriction, hema blood), i.e., insufficient blood supply. The coronary arteries supply the heart with blood and obstruction of coronary blood flow is the most important cause of heart ischemia.

The most common cause of coronary blood flow obstruction is coronary artery disease and the most common coronary artery disease, by far, is atherosclerosis with or without superimposed thrombosis. Atherosclerosis with superimposed thrombosis is called atherothrombosis.

The terms coronary artery disease and ischemic heart disease are sometimes used synonymously because almost all ischemic heart disease is caused by coronary artery disease. However, coronary artery disease is present in asymptomatic individuals for many years before ischemic heart disease develops.

Principally, in heart ischemia all heart tissue types suffer but clinically myocardial ischemia is most important. Myocardial ischemia may lead to myocardial infarction. Acutely, this may lead to heart failure and/or arrhythmia. Chronically, myocardial scar- ring may also cause heart failure and/or arrhythmia.

Key symptoms of myocardial ischemia are chest discomfort and shortness of breath but myocardial ischemia can also be clinically silent.

The first symptom of ischemic heart disease may be sudden death in up to 20 % of cases, stable angina pectoris in 40-50 %, and acute myocardial infarction in 30-40 %.

STABLE ANGINA PECTORIS

Symptoms of myocardial ischemia are brought on when extra heart work is demanded, e.g. by physical exertion or emotional distress. Classically, the symptoms are relieved within minutes by rest and nitroglycerin.

ACUTE CORONARY SYNDROMES

Symptoms of myocardial ischemia usually start abruptly and are not relieved by rest or nitroglycerin. Without evidence of myocardial damage, the condition is referred to as unstable angina. With evidence of myocardial damage, the condition is referred to as acute myocardial infarction.

CULPRIT LESION

The lesion responsible for clinical symptoms, such as an acute coronary syndrome or stable angina pectoris, is called the culprit lesion.

CORONARY ARTERY ATHEROSCLEROSIS

CORONARY ATHEROSCLEROSIS

Atherosclerosis is a chronic immunoinflammatory disease of the intima of medium-sized and large arteries, including the coronary arteries, driven by lipids. Initially, blood lipids enter the intima from the luminal side. Later, a significant contribution to intimal lipids may come from small, fragile vessels entering the intima from the adventitia. Atherosclerosis is multifocal. A focus of atherosclerosis is generally called a lesion and more advanced lesions are often referred to as plaques. Although atherosclerosis primarily is an intimal disease, advanced atherosclerotic plaques are also associated with medial destruction and adventitial vascularization and inflammation.

EXPANSIVE REMODELING, PLAQUE SIZE AND STENOSIS

When a plaque forms, the artery may undergo compensatory enlargement and thereby "make room" for both a large plaque and the lumen. This process is known as expansive remodeling.

Owing to expansive remodeling, a large plaque can be present with only limited luminal narrowing or without narrowing at all. However, not all large plaques are associated with expansive remodeling and these will cause luminal stenosis. A plaque causing stenosis is the most common cause of stable angina.

With expansive remodeling in mind, assessment of the coronary lumen with angiography does not give an accurate assessment of plaques harbored in the artery wall. In vivo assessment of both plaque size and expansive remodeling is possible with both invasive and non-invasive imaging.

CORONARY ARTERY ATHEROTHROMBOSIS

THROMBOSED PLAQUES

A plaque with a superimposed thrombus is called a thrombosed plaque.

Advances in clinical imaging technologies have paved the way for in vivo investigation of thrombosed plaques in acute coronary syndrome patients. Thrombosed plaques have been studied for many years by pathologists, and their studies are the main source of our knowledge about thrombosed plaques. Pathologists utilize an imaging modality with higher resolution than any clinical imaging modality available today, i.e. microscopy.

THROMBOSED PLAQUE TYPES

Based on microscopic examination, thrombosed plaques can be divided into two groups, i.e. ruptured and non-ruptured plaques.

Ruptured plaques have deep injury with a defect or gap in the fibrous cap that separated its lipid-rich atheromatous core from the flowing blood.

Non-ruptured plaques do not have such a deep injury with a defect or gap in their surface. The underlying mechanisms eliciting acute coronary thrombosis in non-ruptured plaques are elusive but the term plaque erosion, suggestive of a mechanism involving endothelial erosion over the plaque, is often used.

Frequency of thrombosed plaque types

Overall, ruptured coronary plaques are responsible for approximately 75 % of fatal and non-fatal coronary thrombi. This makes the ruptured plaque the most important thrombosed plaque type.

CORONARY CONSEQUENCES OF PLAQUE RUPTURE

The fibrous cap is the tissue layer separating a lipid-rich atheromatous core from the blood. Plaque rupture is the process where the deep injury, defect, or gap in the fibrous cap arises.

Consequential to plaque rupture, lipid-rich atheromatous core material may be dislodged into the lumen and embolize to the distal coronary circulation and hemorrhage from the lumen into the plaque, i.e. plaque hemorrhage, may occur. The contents of the lipid-rich atheromatous core are highly thrombogenic, and exposure of the lipid-rich atheromatous core leads to acute coronary thrombosis.

Depending on the thrombogenic stimulus, the coronary flow, and the thrombogenicity of the blood, the thrombus may wax and wane, and lead to varying degrees of coronary flow obstruction up to total obstruction.

A ruptured plaque with superimposed non-occluding thrombus can heal with thrombus incorporation into the plaque. This leads to plaque progression with or without significant stenosis formation.

CLINICAL CONSEQUENCES OF PLAQUE RUPTURE

Plaque rupture followed by thrombosis is the leading cause of the acute coronary syndrome.

Plaque rupture followed by thrombosis and healing may also lead to clinically silent lesion progression or progression to a lesion that causes stenosis and stable angina pectoris.

THE VULNERABLE ATHEROMATOUS PLAQUE

THE VULNERABLE PLAQUE CONCEPT

The vulnerable plaque is the plaque that was present immediately before plaque thrombosis. By inference from the observations of thrombosed plaques, we imagine the appearance of the plaque immediately before plaque thrombosis.

Reliable prospective identification of vulnerable plaques is unproven.

THE VULNERABLE ATHEROMATOUS PLAQUE

The vulnerable atheromatous plaque is the ruptured plaque precursor. This plaque is also called a plaque prone to rupture or a thin-cap fibroatheroma (TCFA).

Since the definition of plaque rupture relies on the presence of a lipid-rich atheromatous core covered by a fibrous cap, these two structures are the key components of the vulnerable atheromatous plaque but other plaque features are also associated with vulnerable atheromatous plaques. Of these, expansive remodeling, intimal microvessels, and calcification are discussed here.

THE   LIPID-RICH ATHEROMATOUS CORE

A large lipid-rich atheromatous core is associated with plaque rupture and covered on average 29-34% of plaque area in ruptured human coronary plaques. The core is lipid-rich and contains free cholesterol.

The core is atheromatous (Greek: athera gruel), i.e. of soft gruel-like substance. The key feature defining the lipid-rich atheromatous core is its lack of supporting collagen. Soft gruel-like and with lack of structural support, an enlarging lipid-rich atheromatous core confers mechanical instability and increasing tensile stress to the overlying fibrous cap and erodes the fibrous cap from below during enlargement.

The lipid-rich atheromatous core is a cellular but it is rich in cellular debris from apoptosis and necrosis of smooth muscle cells and lipid-filled macrophages (foam cells). Since cell death is believed to play an important role in the formation of a lipid-rich core, it is also called a necrotic core which is synonymous with lipid-rich atheromatous core.

THE FIBROUS CAP

The fibrous cap is the tissue layer separating a lipid-rich atheromatous core from the blood. It consists of smooth muscle cells and the extracellular matrix they synthesize (mainly collagen and proteoglycans). The cap also contains inflammatory cells; predominantly macrophage foam cells.

Plaque rupture only occurs when the fibrous cap is extremely thin. In a post mortem series of 41 ruptured coronary plaques, 95 % of the fibrous caps were < 65 µm thick (mean 23 µm). Based on this finding, a thin fibrous cap is usually defined as a cap with a thickness < 65 µm. Recently, a mean fibrous cap thickness of 49 µm in ruptured coronary plaques in patients with acute myocardial infarction was found with in vivo optical coherence tomography.

Thinning of the fibrous cap is considered a product of in- creased matrix degradation by infiltrating macrophages and de- creased matrix synthesis due to a decreasing number of cap smooth muscle cells.

ATHEROSCLEROSIS

Atherosclerosis is characterised by the hardening and narrowing of the arteries, impairing blood flow to the heart and brain caused by the accumulation of atherosclerotic plaque in the arteries. The inner cell lining of the arteries is made up of fat, cholesterol, and other substances found in the blood, called the endothelium. Subsequently, as plaque builds, an inflammatory response from the immune system will cause even more damage to the arteries. A partial or total blockage may occur and stop blood flow through the arteries of the brain, pelvis, heart, legs, arms, or kidneys caused by obstructive plaques. When this happens, the site of the plaque determines the type of coronary disease. These include:

- Coronary heart disease
- Angina
- Carotid artery disease
- Peripheral artery disease
- Chronic kidney disease

During early stages of atherosclerosis, there may be no visible symptoms for several years. You can analogise this to an overlooked plumbing issue with pipes. To get a better idea of things, just imagine a thick sludge forming on the inside of those pipes, creating a large obstruction and blocking anything that tries to pass. It may not be a perfect comparison regarding atherosclerosis, as buildups don't just form on artery walls, but inside them. Still, you get the idea. Eventually, if this disease progresses, it will get to the point where you may feel these symptoms, which can be experienced during activity or at rest:

• Chest pain (This varies for men and women)

• Radiating pain throughout body

• Shortness of breath

• Overwhelming fatigue

• Sweating

• Nausea

• Breathing difficulties

• Heart palpitations

• Loss of consciousness

It's not known what exactly causes atherosclerosis to develop, but smoking cigarettes, high blood pressure, high glucose levels, and high cholesterol levels could possibly contribute to one's risk. For example, when "bad cholesterol" builds up in coronary artery walls, the body will send white blood cells and other cells to the toxic site. Over the years, a bump on the artery wall can develop and obstruct the supply of blood flow. This will eventually cause plaques to form. Patients will take prescribed medication to treat this disease, including blood thinners and statins commonly used to lower cholesterol levels. Although these kinds of medications may be life-saving and prevent future cardiac events, they are moderately effective and not without side effects. These include:

- Prolonged bleeding

- Bleeding gums

- Nosebleeds

- Bloody urine or feces

- Unusually heavy menstruation

Scientific literature has suggested that psychoactive compounds such as THC have a profound influence and beneficial effect on immune system cells. THC is said to decrease secretion of proinflammatory substances and their migration to the artery vessel wall.

Atherosclerosis Signs and Symptoms

You might not have symptoms until your artery is nearly closed or until you have a heart attack or stroke. Signs can also depend on which artery is narrowed or blocked.

Symptoms related to your coronary arteries include:

- Arrhythmia, an unusual heartbeat

- Pain or pressure in your upper body, including your chest, arms, neck, or jaw. This is known as angina.

- Shortness of breath

Symptoms related to the arteries that deliver blood to your brain include:

- Numbness or weakness in your arms or legs

- A hard time speaking or understanding someone who's talking

- Drooping facial muscles

- Paralysis

- Severe headache

- Trouble seeing in one or both eyes

Symptoms related to the arteries of your arms, legs, and pelvis include:

- Leg pain when walking

- Numbness

Symptoms related to the arteries that deliver blood to your kidneys include:

- High blood pressure

- Kidney failure

Atherosclerosis Diagnosis

Your doctor will start with a physical exam. They'll listen to your arteries and check for weak or absent pulses.

You might need tests, including:

• Angiogram, in which your doctor puts dye into your arteries so they'll be visible on an X-ray

• Ankle-brachial index, a test to compare blood pressures in your lower leg and arm

• Blood tests to look for things that raise your risk of having atherosclerosis, like high cholesterol or blood sugar

• Chest X-ray to check for signs of heart failure

• CT scan or magnetic resonance angiography (MRA) to look for hardened or narrowed arteries

• EKG, a record of your heart's electrical activity

• Stress test, in which you exercise while health care professionals watch your heart rate, blood pressure, and breathing

You might also need to see doctors who specialize in certain parts of your body, like cardiologists or vascular specialists, depending on your condition.

Atherosclerosis Causes

Arteries are blood vessels that carry blood from your heart throughout your body. They're lined by a thin layer of cells called the endothelium. It keeps the inside of your arteries in shape and smooth, which keeps blood flowing.

Atherosclerosis begins with damage to the endothelium. Common causes include:

• High cholesterol

• High blood pressure

• Inflammation, like from arthritis or lupus

- Obesity or diabetes

- Smoking

That damage causes plaque to build up along the walls of your arteries.

When bad cholesterol, or LDL, crosses a damaged endothelium, it enters the wall of your artery. Your white blood cells stream in to digest the LDL. Over the years, cholesterol and cells become plaque in the wall of your artery.

Plaque creates a bump on your artery wall. As atherosclerosis gets worse, that bump gets bigger. When it gets big enough, it can create a blockage.

That process goes on throughout your entire body. It's not only your heart at risk. You're also at risk for stroke and other health problems.

Atherosclerosis usually doesn't cause symptoms until you're middle-age or older. As the narrowing becomes severe, it can choke off blood flow and cause pain.

Blockages can also rupture suddenly. That causes blood to clot inside an artery at the site of the rupture.

Atherosclerosis Risk Factors

Atherosclerosis starts when you're young. Research has found that even teenagers can have signs.

If you're 40 and generally healthy, you have about a 50% chance of getting serious atherosclerosis in your lifetime. The risk goes up as you get older. Most adults older than 60 have some atherosclerosis, but most don't have noticeable symptoms.

These risk factors are behind more than 90% of all heart attacks:

• Abdominal obesity ("spare tire")

• Diabetes

• High alcohol intake (more than one drink for women, one or two drinks for men, per day)

- High blood pressure

- High cholesterol

- Not eating fruits and vegetables

- Not exercising regularly

- Smoking

- Stress

Rates of death from atherosclerosis have fallen 25% in the past 3 decades. This is because of better lifestyles and improved treatments.

Plaque Attacks

Plaques from atherosclerosis can behave in different ways.

They can stay in your artery wall. There, the plaque grows to a certain size and then stops. Since this plaque doesn't block blood flow, it may never cause symptoms.

Plaque can grow in a slow, controlled way into the path of blood flow. Over time, it causes significant blockages. Pain in your chest or legs when you exert yourself is the usual symptom.

The worst happens when plaques suddenly rupture, allowing blood to clot inside an artery. In your brain, this causes a stroke; in your heart, a heart attack.

The plaques of atherosclerosis cause the three main kinds of cardiovascular disease:

• Coronary artery disease: Stable plaques in your heart's arteries cause angina (chest pain). Sudden plaque rupture and clotting cause heart muscle to die. This is a heart attack.

• Cerebrovascular disease: Ruptured plaques in your brain's arteries cause strokes with the potential for permanent brain damage. Temporary blockages in your artery can also cause something called transient ischemic attacks (TIAs), which are warning signs of a stroke. They don't cause any brain injury.

• Peripheral artery disease: When the arteries in your legs narrow, it can lead to poor circulation. This makes it painful for you to walk. Wounds also won't heal as well. If you have a severe form of the disease, you might need to have a limb removed (amputation).

Atherosclerosis Complications

Complications of atherosclerosis include:

- Aneurysms

- Angina

- Chronic kidney disease

- Coronary or carotid heart disease

- Heart attack

- Heart failure

- Peripheral artery disease

- Stroke

- Unusual heart rhythms

Atherosclerosis Treatment

Once you have a blockage, it's generally there to stay. But with medication and lifestyle changes, you can slow or stop plaques. They may even shrink slightly with aggressive treatment.

Lifestyle changes: You can slow or stop atherosclerosis by taking care of the risk factors. That means a healthy diet, exercise, and no smoking. These changes won't remove blockages, but they're proven to lower the risk of heart attacks and strokes.

Medication: Drugs for high cholesterol and high blood pressure will slow and may even halt atherosclerosis. They could also lower your risk of hearts attack and strokes.

Your doctor can use more invasive techniques to open blockages from atherosclerosis or go around them:

- Angiography and stenting: Your doctor puts a thin tube into an artery in your leg or arm to get to diseased arteries. Blockages are visible on a live X-ray screen. Angioplasty (using a catheter with a balloon tip) and stenting can often open a blocked artery. Stenting helps ease symptoms, but it does not prevent heart attacks.

• **Bypass surgery**: Your doctor takes a healthy blood vessel, often from your leg or chest, and uses it to go around a blocked segment.

• **Endarterectomy**: Your doctor goes into the arteries in your neck to remove plaque and restore blood flow.

• **Fibrinolytic therapy:** A drug dissolves a blood clot that's blocking your artery.

CANNABINOIDS AND ATHEROSCLEROSIS

To determine the role of marijuana in atherosclerotic coronary heart disease prevention, we must first understand how cannabinoid receptors work in the endocannabinoid system. The endocannabinoid system is comprised of cannabinoids and plays a vital role in maintaining proper cell function in different systems of the body. Basically, there are two main cell receptors that make up the ECS: Cannabinoid Receptor 1 and Cannabinoid Receptor 2. CB1 receptors are found mostly on brain cells and are responsible for the chemical's psychotropic effects, while CB2 receptors are more abundant and mostly found on immune cells.

There are many cannabinoid receptors found on the surface of cells in the human body. Major organs like the brain, heart, liver, and vascular smooth muscle cells (VSMCs) have CB1 receptors. Small, naturally-produced fat-like molecules within cell membranes known as endocannabinoids, endo meaning "within", activate these receptors and act as the body's natural THC. Endocannabinoids are synthesised on-demand; in other words, they get made and used exactly when they're needed, rather than being stored away for later use like many other biological molecules in the body.

When cannabis is consumed, psychoactive compound THC interacts with CB1 and CB2 receptors. Immediately, cannabinoids bind to CB2 receptors and fight atherosclerosis by producing changes in brain messages and also by regulating blood circulation and cardiac functions.

TESTING THC ON MICE

A study conducted by Francois Mach and colleagues showed that cannabis compounds are beneficial to blood vessels and reduced progression of atherosclerosis in mice. In the study, a group of mice were given a high cholesterol diet for 11 weeks, designed to clog their arteries. Halfway through the diet at 6 weeks, some mice were orally administered 1 mg of THC daily, which yielded the most significant improvements.

Predominant psychoactive compound THC was shown to inhibit disease progression through pleiotropic effects (which statins also accomplish) on inflammatory cells. Afterwards, findings revealed that mice who had received THC had a lower level of blood vessel clogging than the others. When another drug was used to block CB2 receptors in the mice, THC couldn't prevent buildup from fatty deposits in the animals' arteries. As for the CB1 receptors, the THC dose orally administered in the study was in an amount that was not high enough to actually produce psychoactive effects. During treatment, not one mouse showed unhealthy behavior. According to researchers of the cardiology division at University Hospital in Geneva, Switzerland including Mach, the results may be due to THC's anti-inflammatory properties. Dr. Mach believes future work regarding cannabis and inflammatory diseases will focus on finding drugs that mimic the benefit without producing the effects of cannabis on the brain.

FINAL THOUGHTS

Perhaps there is more research needed on the use of cannabis and preventing coronary diseases. The recreational use of cannabis may not be the best way to benefit from the plant's medicinal properties. In other studies, it's been found that cannabis use increased the risk of coronary and cardiovascular complications. Consuming marijuana increases heart rate and standing blood pressure, and also reduces lying blood pressure. This is why medical marijuana is suggested, as studies also show that various cannabinoids have their own effects on atherosclerosis.

Luckily, there is still hope for those wanting to naturally regulate and prevent problems caused by arterial plaque without traditional pharmaceuticals. Doctors have been prescribing patients edibles and vaporizers, as it is said to be a safer and healthier way to consume cannabis, especially for patients who are already sick. There are also some lifestyle changes a patient can make to manage atherosclerosis. It is important to:

• Get your cholesterol regularly checked

• Eat a low-saturated fat, low-cholesterol, and low-sodium diet

• Exercise regularly

• Maintain a healthy weight to reduce risk factors such as high blood pressure

ATHEROSCLEROSIS: A COMPLETE OVERVIEW OF THE DISEASE

Atherosclerosis is the narrowing and hardening of the arteries. It impairs the flow of blood to the brain and the heart which is caused due to the build-up of atherosclerotic plaque (build-up of lipids within the arterial wall). This continues to accumulate in the arteries. Cholesterol, fat, and several other substances present in the blood from the inner lining of the arteries. However, as an atherosclerotic plaque continues to form, the immune system responds by inducing inflammation, which will result in way more damage. A total or partial blockage can occur which will stop the flow of blood through different arteries of the pelvis, brain, legs, arms, kidneys, or heart due to the obstructive plaques.

Early stages of this disease don't bring with it any kind of visible symptoms. The build-up continues to form inside the artery walls and gradually these symptoms can be experienced.

Radiating pain, Chest pain, Overwhelming fatigue, Shortness of breath, Nausea, Sweating, Heart palpitations, Breathing difficulties, Loss of consciousness; any of these symptoms may be experienced according to the site of occurrence of the atherosclerotic plaque.

Scientific studies conducted over the years have suggested that the psychoactive compounds present in cannabis i.e. Tetrahydrocannabinol (THC) can have a beneficial effect on the immune system cells. THC can decrease proinflammatory substances secretion and the migration of these substances to the vessel wall.

How Cannabis Influences Atherosclerosis?

In order to understand the role that cannabis plays in the prevention of coronary heart disease, we need to understand how the cannabinoid receptors function in the whole endocannabinoid system (ECS). Comprised of cannabinoids the endocannabinoid system plays a primary role in the maintenance of proper cell function occurring in the different systems of your body.

The current body of evidence supporting a therapeutic role for CBD in cardiovascular disorders

There are two primary cell receptors that make the ECS :

- Cannabinoid Receptor 1 (CB1)

- Cannabinoid Receptor 2 (CB2)

CB1 receptors are present in the brain cells. They are responsible for chemical psychotropic effects whereas the CB2 receptors are abundant and found in the immune cells. All the major organs – heart, brain, liver, and VSMCs (Vascular Smooth

Muscle Cells) have CB1 receptors. Endocannabinoids are the naturally produced, small molecules present within the cell membranes. You will be amazed to know that endocannabinoids are synthesized every time they are needed. They aren't stored for later use. Upon the consumption of cannabis, THC (the psychoactive compound) reacts with both receptors (CB1 and CB2). This is done by producing a change in the brain messages as well as regulating cardiac functions and blood circulations.

The pharmacologic effects of cannabinoids, based on their interaction with cannabinoid receptors (CB1 and CB2), which are widely distributed in the cardiovascular system, have been well described. Activation of these receptors modulates the function of various cellular components of the vessel wall and may contribute to the pathogenesis of atherosclerosis.

The role of CB2 receptor activation on atherosclerosis occurrence has been studied and it was shown that CB2 stimulation leads to attenuation of the inflammatory response in the pathogenesis of atherosclerosis. Various investigations on models of human diseases support the idea that CBD lessens the inflammation beyond the known antioxidant properties of CBD. The therapeutic utility of CBD is a relatively new area of investigation that will result in new discoveries on the interaction between inflammation and oxidative stress and the endocannabinoid system (ECS), a relationship that highlights the tissue and organ damage in many human disorders, including atherosclerosis.

CBD OIL FOR ATHEROSCLEROSIS

CBD can be an effective and safe therapeutic aid for atherosclerosis because it reduces myocardial ischemic. Atherosclerosis, or hardening of arteries, occurs when vessels become thick and rigid. Arteries can also be damaged due to a metabolic disorder, or the aging process. Substances like proteins, calcium, and lipids are slowly deposited throughout the body's circulation system. Eventually, this life threatening disorder can occur. Nevertheless, this severe condition can be prevented and potentially relieved with the help of CBD.

It's important to note that the severe heart condition is among the major causes of death in America. Currently, the severe condition causes more deaths than cancer. Seventy-five percent of cardiovascular related deaths are caused by atherosclerosis, despite the fact that the condition can potentially be relieved.

HOW CBD HELPS WITH ATHEROSCLEROSIS

Cannabinoid receptors in the cardiovascular system play a crucial role in the regulation of circulation and heart function. Body cannabinoids and CBD are the major regulators of the immune-inflammation system and circulatory functions. Since atherosclerosis is largely characterized by inflammation, researchers suggest that the use of CBD can counter the severe condition's progression.

Basically, cannabidiol or CBD, can act as an immunomodulating agent. That means it can be used to lessen atherosclerosis progression especially when the severe condition is caused by a high glucose level. It can also help in fighting the severe condition known as ischemia. This is a harmful metabolic syndrome complication. Several human and animal studies have indicated that using CBD to activate CB2 receptors can reduce several endothelial-related and circulatory issues.

HOW CANNABIDIOL WORKS

CBD causes blood vessels to widen and relax. It has been proven effective in protecting the integrity of the endothelial cells in the coronary artery and their overall endothelial function. CBD has also been proven effective in reducing cardiac fibrosis, myocardial dysfunction, inflammation, cell death, oxidative-nitrative stress, and inter-related signaling pathways. All these provide therapeutic benefits to individuals that suffer from atherosclerosis.

Administration of CBD immediately after a person suffers a heart attack has been proven effective in the reduction of infarct size as well as myocardial inflammation. This shows that CBD can be a very effective therapeutic aid for myocardial ischemia.

WHEN CHOOSING TO USE CBD FOR ATHEROSCLEROSIS RELIEF SUPPLEMENT

Atherosclerosis patients that want to use CBD as a therapeutic aid should talk to their doctor first. A licensed doctor should evaluate the file of the patient and provide a recommendation on whether CBD can be used or not. Nevertheless, we have a wide range of CBD product articles to give you all the information you need before choosing a cannabidiol product to relieve atherosclerosis. They include CBD edibles, CBD gummies, CBD oil, CBD drip and crystals among others. Simply browse through our articles to learn more about the best CBD product for you or your loved ones.

SUMMARY

Advanced atherosclerosis, through thrombosis, leads to ischemic heart disease and ischemic stroke, the leading causes of death and disability worldwide. Advanced atherosclerosis and imaging of atherosclerosis are the focus of this dissertation with particular emphasis on the vulnerable plaque and vulnerable plaque detection. Aspects of advanced atherosclerosis and the vulnerable plaque in humans are described along with the basis for the selected minipig models and methods for atherosclerosis acceleration used. The overall aims of the studies were to develop an animal model of advanced atherosclerosis with human-like vulnerable plaque morphology and use this animal model to test an imaging modality aimed at vulnerable plaque detection. The first aim is addressed in 3 papers, where accelerated plaque development in the coronary and carotid arteries is investigated in down-sized Rapacz pigs.

Down-sized Rapacz pigs are minipigs with familial hypercholesterolemia caused by a mutation in the low density lipoprotein receptor. Paper 1 describes the lipid profile in the down-sized Rapacz on chow and atherogenic diets and spontaneously developed and balloon-accelerated coronary plaque with a morphology that resembles the morphology of human vulnerable plaque. Paper 2 describes vein graft disease in internal jugular vein grafts inserted into the common carotid artery. Plaques with necrotic cores were found in oversized vein grafts only indicating an effect of flow and shear stress on plaque development. Paper 3 describes the effects of wall shear stress on local plaque development in surgically stenosed common carotid arteries in the down-sized Rapacz pigs. This study indicated that the com- bination of low and oscillatory wall shear stress was needed for development of advanced plaque. In paper 4, we interrogated coronary lesions in the down-sized Rapacz with a commercially available diagnostic tool VH IVUS. It is claimed that VH IVUS can characterize the tissue com- ponents that constitute plaque reliably. However, we found that VH IVUS does not reliably assess the most important plaque com- ponent of all, i.e. the necrotic core. In conclusion, we developed an animal model of advanced atherosclerosis with human-like vulnerable plaque morphology. The usefulness of this animal model was demonstrated in a study testing an imaging modality aimed at vulnerable plaque detection in humans.

CONCLUSION

In summary, this review has presented evidence of the positive effects of CBD in the cardiovascular system, summarised in isolated arteries, direct application of CBD causes both acute and time-dependent vasorelaxation of preconstricted arteries and enhances endothelium-dependent vasorelaxation in models of endothelial dysfunction. In vivo, CBD treatment does not appear to have any effect on resting blood pressure or heart rate, but does reduce the cardiovascular response to various types of stress. In vivo, CBD treatment has a protective role in reducing the effects of cardiac ischaemia and reperfusion, or in reducing cardiac dysfunction associated with diabetes. Similarly, CBD has a protective role in reducing the ischaemic damage in models of stroke, partly due to maintaining cerebral blood flow. In models of altered vascular permeability, CBD reduces the hyperpermeability of the BRB in diabetes and BBB hyperpermeability after LPS injection. Similarly, CBD ameliorates the negative effects of a high glucose environment on cell adhesion molecules and barrier function. Together, these data suggest that the cardiovascular system is indeed a valid therapeutic target for CBD. However, the target sites of action for CBD remain to be established for most of these responses. Whether these responses to CBD will translate into the human cardiovascular system also remains to be established.

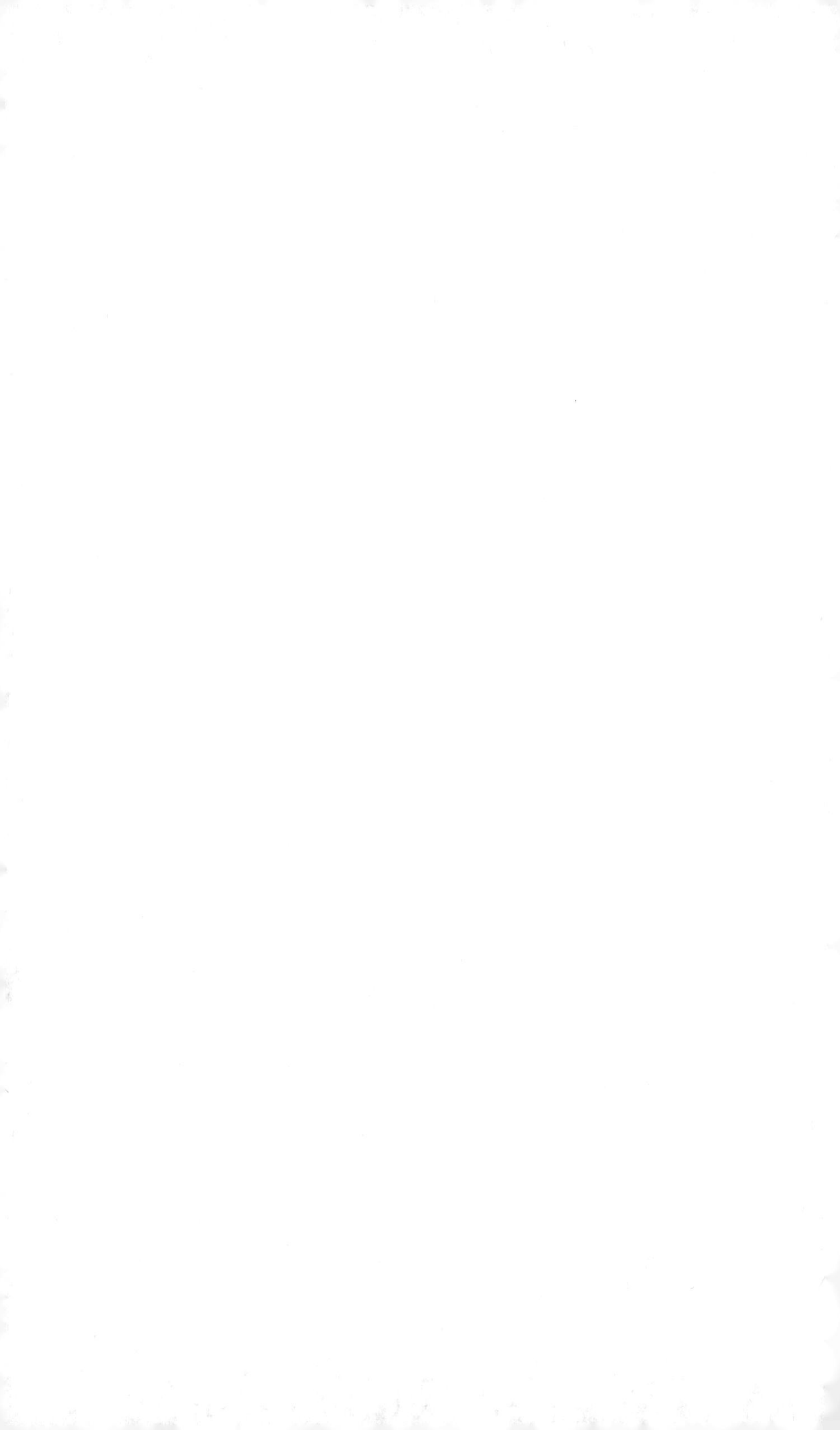

www.ingramcontent.com/pod-product-compliance
Lightning Source LLC
Chambersburg PA
CBHW061739250726
48657CB00002B/1001